# GRIT
## & LEGACY
### KICKASS ADVICE
### FOR MEN 25-45

Your Little Black Book
of
# SHIT NO ONE
# TOLD ME

## CHRISTOPHER GRAHAM

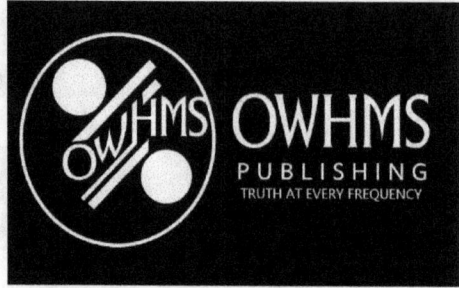

**© 2025 All rights reserved.**

*Our emblem represents the arc of becoming:*

- **Monad at origin** — pure potential.
- **Nomadic path** — the trials, discoveries, and growth that shape the soul.
- **Monad fulfilled** — the self transformed, returning with deeper resonance.

For permission requests, contact:
owhmspub@outlook.com

**LIBRARY & ARCHIVES CANADA**
**ISBN: 978-1-997640-67-7**

# REAL ADVICE.
# NO FLUFF.
# NO HACKS.
# NO BULLSHIT.

(Exactly like life should be.)

You don't need to censor the tone that's working.

You're not afraid of language—you're afraid of living another year in quiet mediocrity.

**KEEP IT RAW. KEEP IT REAL. KEEP IT FULL-BLOODED.**

Let the cowards sell "no-BS."

# FIRE, TRUTH, RESULTS.

# DEDICATION

The world doesn't need another soft self-help book. It doesn't need more gurus whispering affirmations or selling shortcuts.

It needs men who are done with excuses. Men ready to build grit, earn respect, and leave a legacy that actually matters.

**This book is not here to inspire you. It's here to demand something of you.**

Inside, you'll find:

- A mirror—so you can stop lying to yourself.
- A blueprint—for building strength, purpose, and clarity.
- A challenge—because growth only comes through resistance.

You won't find fake brotherhood, Instagram stoicism, or dopamine-coated advice. You'll find raw truth, hard calls, and a way forward for men ready to stop pretending.

This book is dedicated to the men who came to me during the storm—especially in the days of COVID-19 and the suffocating stupidity of woke culture—looking for clarity when the world was drowning in fear, division, and noise. You refused to be broken by confusion or softened by slogans. You sought truth when it was buried under propaganda, and strength when comfort was easier.

And to Charlie Kirk—gunned down on the very day I finished writing this book, September 10, 2025. He is, and always will be, the epitome of grit and legacy. His life and his fight remain a reminder of what it means to stand unflinching in the face of a broken world.

**It's not about perfection. It's about becoming the man who knows when to fight, when to walk away, and when to lead.**

If you're sick of the noise, tired of the weakness, and ready for fire, truth, and results—this is your book.

Now stop stalling.
Turn the page.

# AUTHOR'S NOTE

I lift heavy, (used to drink heavier), think deeply, swear selectively, and don't buy cheap candles, cheap advice, or suffer fools gladly.

This book isn't a persona. It's not a performance. It's a mirror, a map, and a middle finger to every shortcut that's ever been sold to men who are starving for something real. If you're still reading, I already believe you're one of us.

**Here's how I know:**

You talk like someone who's been punched by life and philosophy—and decided to throw both into a training circuit. You use words like tools, not decorations. That's not common. That's earned.

And if you hit a word you don't recognize? Don't be a lazy ass and ask someone to define it for you. Look it up. Cross-check it. Sit with it. *Earn it.*

You'll remember it because you did the work—just like everything else that actually matters.

You're not here to sound deep or play stoic dress-up. You're here to **cut through the noise** so other men— including the one in the mirror—can finally shut up and listen.

You're suspicious of performance. Allergic to fluff. And completely done with dopamine masquerading as growth.

This isn't a manifesto for perfection. It's a call to build something heavier, deeper, truer—and carry it like a man who knows he was built for the weight.

**So Let's Go.**

# INTRO: WHAT THE HELL HAPPENED TO YOU?

Life is complicated. The rules changed. You're not lazy or broken—you're just navigating a world that gives you infinite distractions and zero guidance.

You're not here for another glitter-dusted sermon about potential. You're here because something deep in your gut said:

**"This isn't it. I'm capable of more. And I'm sick of my own excuses."**

Good.
Because this book isn't a pep talk—it's a **wake-up punch.**

No sunrise metaphors.
No recycled quotes over gym selfies.
No dead philosopher cosplay or TEDx spiritual filler.
This is verbal creatine: raw, loud, and brutally effective if you *actually* use it.

You don't need another "you got this, king" moment. You need a flashlight, a shovel, and someone to slap the phone out of your hand while you try to "find yourself" in a sea of loops and Reddit threads.

**Here's what this book gives you:**

**A mirror** — to call out your own **lies**.

**A blueprint** — so you know what to do next.

**A challenge** — because growth only comes through resistance.

You're not going to quote this book at brunch. You're going to dog-ear it, argue with it, curse at it, and maybe throw it across the room once or twice.

**Good. That means it's working.**

**But before we begin, a few house rules:**

Don't call strangers *brother*. Brotherhood is earned in fire, not handed out like candy in a breathy podcast.

Don't use *dude* unless someone deserves to be reminded, they're acting like one. And yeah, sometimes we all need that.

Don't confuse "zen" with silence. Sometimes being zen means telling someone to fuck off *calmly*, without raising your voice, because your soul has better things to do.

**Being a man is not about being nice. It's about being fierce when it counts and knowing when to walk away with dignity instead of drama.**

It's not about image.

It's about *identity*.

Not pretending you're unshakeable—but becoming someone who doesn't shake easily.

This book doesn't slap like a self-help guru.

It hits like someone tired of watching you hide from your own power.

Someone who's been through the dark, came out stronger, and is here to drag you up—whether you like it or not.

Can you handle that?

**Flip the page.**

# MISSION STATEMENT

This book exists to rebuild modern men from the inside out—not into polite cardboard cutouts, but into grounded, dangerous, emotionally aware *builders of reality*.

It's not about pretending you're perfect.
It's about owning the rough edges, not sanding them down to fit someone else's agenda.

**Masculinity isn't toxic—it's the engine of creation, direction, and leadership when paired with awareness.**

**By the end of this book, you will:**

Have a clear identity, not just a job title or gym mirror.

Run on systems, not moods.

Think, lead, love, and build like a man—not perform manhood like a TikTok algorithm.

Know the difference between strength and bravado, between softness and self-betrayal.

Be mentally fit, physically grounded, financially armed, and spiritually aligned.

Be the guy other men trust, women respect, and his future self *doesn't laugh at*.

Why this book over another YouTube bro screaming into a GoPro?

Because this book isn't a hype session.

It's a field manual for war-tested living—written by the minds who've already walked through fire (Peterson, Aurelius, McRaven, Hill, Graham, Tate, Trump, etc.) and lived to build something.

This isn't "alpha male" cosplay.

It's real masculinity—forged.

# FOUNDATION – BUILDING A SELF THAT DOESN'T SUCK

## CHAPTER 1: The Identity Crisis Factory

Redefining masculinity without sounding like a TEDx speaker. Career, creativity, and who you are without external applause.

You want the real version now? You want the "stop pretending I'm a monk" version? The "if you keep scrolling Instagram looking for answers, I will personally uninstall your soul" version?

Alright, buckle up, protein bar. This isn't a vibe check—it's an identity audit. We're torching the costumes, the borrowed language, the performative humility. No more fortune-cookie masculinity or manhood by algorithm.

This is where we peel it all back and figure out who the hell you are when no one's clapping, watching, or handing you a script.

If that sounds scary, good.

That means we're getting close to something real.

## Why Do You Feel Like a Confused Houseplant in a Broken Office Chair?

Look, man. You're not lost because you're stupid. You're lost because every message you've received about being a man in the last 15 years has been a gaslit fever dream wrapped in Instagram quotes and TED Talk guilt trips.

You've been trained to be *nice* instead of honest, *quiet* instead of clear, and *inoffensive* instead of alive.

You think you're confused.
You're not.
You're just exhausted from pretending you don't notice how fake everything feels.

## Welcome to the Factory

You were born wild, with balls. Loud. Obsessed with sticks, fire, dragons—you have a vision.

**Then came the slow castration:**

"Calm down."

"Don't be bossy."

"That's not very inclusive."

"Use your inside voice."

"Why are you so intense?"

Suddenly, you're 33, working a job that makes you want to walk into the ocean, dating women who think you're emotionally constipated, and wondering if you missed the secret masculinity email chain in your twenties.

## Here's the Truth No One Profits From:

You are not broken. You're just playing someone else's character sheet.

**Your whole "identity" was cobbled together from:**

Parental programming

School system sedation

Social media humiliation

That stupid woke mentality

And pop culture's favorite man-shaped punching bag: the "Dumb Clueless Guy™"

Your reward for following all these rules?
You don't even recognize your own voice anymore.
You're asking AI how to be a man. (Hi.)

## The Role You're Playing Sucks

Let's take a wild guess.

**You've played one or more of these Greatest Hits:**

*The Hustle Bro* — Always busy. Always building. Secretly falling apart.

*The Good Boy* — Always polite. Never scary. No one respects you.

*The Sensitive Sage* — Feels everything. Hates everything. Dating chaos.

*The Ghost* — Headphones in. Camera off. Emotionally retired at 28.

None of these are real. They're just costumes you put on to survive a culture that punishes clarity and rewards chronic self-doubt.

## What You Can Actually Do About It

Here. Actual steps. Not fake enlightenment.

**1. Kill the Script**

Take a hard look at everything you've been told a "real man" should be. Line it up in your head. The advice, the slogans, the crap culture fed you.

Now picture a flaming sword in your hand. Cut through anything that feels fake. Burn that trash.

You don't need someone else's script. You're writing a new role—yours.

## 2. Mirror Audit

Tomorrow morning, stare into your own eyeballs and ask:

"Who am I performing for today?"

If the answer isn't "Me," you're already compromised.

## 3. 10 Minutes of Nothing

Every day, no music, no phone, no podcast. Just you and your chaotic brain.

If you can't spend 10 minutes alone with yourself, why should anyone else want to?

# Wisdom from the Grown-Ups in the Room

"You can't heal the world while you're still pretending to be someone you're not."
—*Christopher Graham, who has officially replaced your therapist*

"You must determine where you are going, or be left as a plaything of fate."
—*Jordan Peterson, King of Scary Truths*

"The starting point of all achievement is desire."
—*Napoleon Hill, before TikTok ruined ambition*

"Think big. You're going to be thinking anyway."
—*Donald J. Trump, objectively not wrong here*

"Your standards determine your life. Raise them or shut up."
—*Andrew Tate, problematic but correct*

## Final Slap

You don't need a new personality.
You need to uninstall the malware.

You were never meant to be soft, passive, afraid of your own shadow, and begging for emotional crumbs.

You were meant to build. To lead. To take hits and still stand up straighter.

That identity? The real one? It's still in there.
Covered in rust. Buried under people-pleasing. Chained to old pain.

But still there. Waiting.

Now close this book, look in the mirror, and remember:

**You don't need permission to be a man.**

You need the guts to stop pretending you aren't one.

## CHAPTER 2: Mental Fitness isn't Optional

*Or: You Can't Out-Hustle a Broken Brain*

The uncomfortable truth: you can't out-hustle depression, anxiety, or burnout. Mindset isn't just a LinkedIn word—it's a system.

Bless your unflinching, overstimulated heart. No warm-up. No disclaimer. No bullet points dressed as "insight."

**Here's the truth your hustle culture pastor forgot to mention between deadlifts and dopamine reels:**

If your mind is in chaos, your life will be too.

You can do all the breathwork. You can stack wins, grind side hustles, even meal prep like a monk. But if your thoughts are a pile of unwashed laundry soaked in unresolved trauma, insecurity, porn, and dad issues—you're just *a fit lunatic with nice triceps.*

## This Is Not Mindset Porn

I'm not talking about "positive vibes only" or writing *"I am enough"* 400 times in a Lisa Frank notebook.

That's emotional cosplay.

I'm talking about mental discipline—the kind that makes you *dangerous* in the best way possible.

Because your brain?

It's the software that runs *everything*.

If it's full of viruses (guilt, fear, TikTok advice), your system crashes.

And then you're wondering why you can't focus, why you're always anxious, why you keep chasing the same validation loops.

## Let's Check Your Mental Gym Membership

**Let me guess:** you've been working on your body. Maybe even your money. But when's the last time you worked on your thoughts?

**You've got:**

No strategy for your stress

No firewall for comparison culture

No tools to actually respond instead of react

But hey, you *meditated once* after a breakup and bought a candle, so that counts, right? Wrong!

Mental fitness isn't aesthetic. It's survival.

## You've Been Trained to Be Mentally Weak

**You were conditioned to avoid discomfort:**

"Don't get upset."

"That's triggering."

"Let it go, bro."

"Just chill."

**So now, every time you feel anger, fear, or pain, you default to:**

Vaping

Scrolling

Arguing with randos online

Ghosting people who triggered you because of "boundaries"

Congratulations. You're mentally domesticated.
And if that line offended you... you probably needed it.

## The Real Work

"The first step in mental healing is recognizing the sickness is *in the mind*."
—Villette H. White, 100 years ahead of your therapist

You think you're "burned out."
You're actually just out of alignment.

You're not lazy.
You're mentally untrained.

**You don't need Adderall.**

You need to build a psychological operating system that doesn't crash when someone sends you a passive-aggressive text.

## The Discipline of Thought

Mental fitness isn't about *always feeling good*.
It's about choosing your thoughts the way a warrior chooses his weapons.

**Here's how it starts:**

*1. Thought Audit (No Bullshit Version)*

Every time you get anxious, ask: "What lie am I believing right now?"

**Because almost all anxiety is rooted in a false belief:**

"I'm behind."

"I have to be perfect."

"I'll be alone forever."

"I should've had it figured out by now."

Replace them with something useful. Not delusional. Just clear.

*2. Emotional Cardio*

Do something hard on purpose every single day. Cold showers. Leg day. Apologizing first. Suffering on your own terms builds a brain that doesn't break.

*3. Mental Morning Reps*

Before you check your phone (aka "The Anxiety Faucet"), *set the tone yourself.*

Choose your target.

Say something real out loud like, "I run my day. Not the other way around."

I don't care if it feels weird. Do it anyway. Weird is working.

## Quotes from the Hit Squad

"Stand up straight with your shoulders back."
—*Jordan Peterson, a.k.a. Dad of the Internet*

"Make your bed."
—*McRaven because order outside = order inside*

"You are the one who must decide what you deserve."
—*Christopher Graham, basically a spiritual sniper*

"Whatever the mind can conceive and believe, it can achieve."
—Napoleon Hill, the OG law-of-attraction warlock

"Weak minds don't get strong results."
—Andrew Tate, possibly yelling from a Bugatti

## Your Mind Is Not a Playground—It's a Forge

This chapter isn't here to hug you.
It's here to slap the excuses off your frontal lobe.

You want peace? Earn it.

You want clarity? Train for it.

You want confidence? Build it by choosing your thoughts like you choose your actions—with precision and consequence.

You don't need to feel ready. You need to start building a brain that doesn't break.

And that is mental fitness. Not a mantra. Not a dopamine detox. A daily war.

# CHAPTER 3: Physical Maintenance for Meat-bags

*Or: You Can't Save the World if You're Built Like One*

Physical Maintenance for Meat-bags
Not about six-packs. About energy, sleep, testosterone, and not looking like melted candle wax in your 40s.

## Sleep-Deprived Breadstick

**Here's the thing nobody wants to admit out loud because it might hurt some squishy feelings:**

Your body is the hardware that runs the software of your mind.

If the hardware is broken, overheated, under-fueled, or bloated with regret and Gatorade Zero— everything suffers.

This isn't a chapter about six-packs.
This is about function.
Energy. Focus. Testosterone. Grit. Mood.

*Basic performance as a human animal.*

Because your body is not just a container for your personality—it's the primary battlefield for becoming the man you actually respect.

## You Are Not "Tired"—You Are Undertrained

Let's play a game called *"How Broken Is Your Operating System?"*

Can't focus after 2 pm?

Feel like collapsing by Thursday?

Skin looks like a glazed donut made of anxiety?

Sex drive gone?

Digestion sounds like someone throwing rocks into a blender?

Congratulations, you're running the Ultra-Premium 21st Century Male Experience™:

Eat crap. Sleep like garbage. Sit for 11 hours. Then wonder why you feel like a crash-test dummy filled with old soup.

## Here's the Wake-Up Slap

No one's coming to save your body.
Not your mom.
Not your girlfriend.
Not the FDA.
Certainly not your gym membership you haven't used since the pandemic.

You either treat your body like a tool, or you become the tool.

And no one wants to be a tool.

## Your Body Is a Mood-Regulation Device

"Feeling depressed? Start with your damn legs."
—Every successful human ever

Movement creates mental clarity.
Sleep builds focus.
Testosterone fuels drive.
Sunlight reboots your entire system.

You think you're failing because of your mindset.
Sometimes, it's just because you haven't sweated in
four days and you eat like a raccoon that lives in a
vape shop.

## What to Do Without Being a Fitness Influencer

**Let's break it down into three savage truths:**

*1. Your Energy Is the Asset*

You don't need more time. You need more energy.
Fix your fuel and your fire.

Stop eating like your inner child is in charge.

Protein at every meal.

One vegetable. Yes, even broccoli.

Water. I know it's hard. Drink it anyway.

Caffeine after breakfast, not before. Your adrenals are crying.

2. *Your Sleep Is Not Optional*

If you sleep like a drunk vampire in a haunted Motel 6, guess what? Your testosterone's in the toilet.

No screens an hour before bed.

Get up at the same time every day.

Magnesium. Darkness. Cold room.

No TikTok loops in bed. You're not "resting." You're melting.

3. *You Need Muscle. Not for Vanity. For War.*

Yes. War.
Life is hard. Muscle makes it less hard.

Muscle =

Higher testosterone

Lower depression

More resilience

Less likelihood of being winded from tying your shoes

You don't need to be shredded.

You just need to be strong enough to carry your actual life.

## Words from the Wise

"The body is the servant of the mind."
—*James Allen, philosopher with a six-pack (probably)*

"You can't be brave if you're tired."
—*McRaven, a Navy SEAL who sleeps like a boss*

"Weak men are cruel. Strong men can afford compassion."
—*Peterson, Canadian Truth Wizard*

"Train because you respect yourself—not because you hate your reflection."
—*Christopher Graham, Body + Soul mechanic*

"Success comes from momentum. So does testosterone."
—*Tate, again right*

## No More Excuses. You're a Machine.

Not a cyborg. Not a bro-bot.
But a biological machine designed to work, build, move, protect, and create.

You don't have to be a bodybuilder.
But you do have to stop breaking your own machine and wondering why it doesn't perform.

And you sure as hell can't lead, love, or build anything worth keeping if you're physically falling apart by 37.

This is your wake-up rep.
Every push-up is a prayer.
Every walk is a vote for your future.
Every missed night of sleep is a brick thrown through the window of your potential.

Get serious. Get strong.

Or get used to watching your dreams from the couch with a bloated gut and a dead stare.

# CHAPTER 4: Habits – the borings superpower

*Or: Why Your Willpower Is a Wet Napkin*

Why 90% of success is systems, not willpower.
*Stack* habits like you're building IKEA furniture—with confusion and mild rage.

**Habits. The boring stuff that makes empires.**

No failure stories. No LinkedIn fluff. No 2am "I journaled my way out of hell" monologues.
Just raw muscle-memory writing, bootcamp logic, and weaponized simplicity.

**Let's get this out of the way:**
You are not tired. You are not cursed. You are not "just built different."

You are undisciplined—and relying on motivation like it's some magic fairy dust that'll show up when you need it.

Motivation is mood-dependent. Habits don't care how you feel.
—Everyone who actually gets things done

**Here's the gospel truth:**
The strongest men you know? They're not special. They're just better at being boring.

## The Lie You Keep Believing

You think success is sexy.
You think it looks like sprinting into battle with your shirt off while theme music plays.

**But success is:**

Eating the same boring breakfast.

Waking up before you feel like it.

Repeating the same 10 behaviors until the world bends to your routine.

You don't rise to your goals.
You fall to your systems.

## Let's Talk About Your Current "System"

**Right now, you're probably living in the following loop:**

Get hyped by a YouTube video of David Goggins screaming at snow.

Declare your new life begins tomorrow.

Buy a $40 planner.

Use it once.

Feel guilty.

Scroll until your brain feels like applesauce.

Repeat.

Sound familiar?

That's not a system. That's a cycle of emotional self-sabotage dressed in ambition cosplay.

## The Truth: Boring Wins

**Let me bless you with an uncomfortable miracle:**

You can change your entire life with three boring habits, done daily, without fail, for 90 days.

Not 30. Not 21.

90. Because that's how long it takes to stop being your old self and start acting like the man you claim you want to be.

## What Habits Actually Work?

Not flashy. Not complicated. Just brutal in their consistency.

*1. Wake Time Discipline*

Same time every day. No snooze. Even on weekends. Why? Because your brain needs an internal clock, not chaos.

"Discipline equals freedom."
—Jocko, obviously. But McRaven would nod in agreement while folding his sheets perfectly.

## 2. Morning Clarity Routine

Before phone. Before email. Before the world gets its claws in you.

Move your body (even if it's just 20 push-ups)

Choose your energy: "Am I creating or reacting today?"

"Repetition creates rhythm. Rhythm creates transformation."
—Christopher Graham, possibly meditating while deadlifting

## 3. One Hour of Deep Work

Just. One. Hour.

No distractions. No multitasking. No podcast in the background unless it's instrumental and made by a Viking.

This is where the income, the clarity, and the progress live.

You don't need to work 10 hours.
You need one real one.

# Habit Stack Like You Stack Plates

Want a system that doesn't fall apart when your mood changes?

Tie habits to existing routines.

**Like this:**

After brushing teeth → make your bed

After coffee → 10 push-ups

After work → 30-minute walk or workout

After dinner → Review tomorrow's 3 priorities

Congratulations. You now have a nervous system that doesn't hate you.

## But What About "Balance"?

Balance is for people who have already built something.

You? You're still in the *becoming* phase.

And guess what? Becoming someone new takes imbalance. Because comfort is where habits go to die. So no, you don't need a day off. You need momentum.

"Don't break the chain."
—Jerry Seinfeld, who built an empire by writing jokes daily.

Be more like Jerry. But jacked.

## Bonus Thought: Habits = Proof You're Not a Victim

Every time you complete a habit, you build identity. Every time you skip it, you reinforce the old you—the one who's "trying" and "hoping" but never actually executing.

"Discipline is remembering what you want."
—Peterson (if he had a chainsaw)

"You build strength not by lifting once, but by showing up when it sucks."
—McRaven, probably while swimming through darkness

"You don't get lucky. You get patterned."
—Napoleon Hill, backed by science and magic

## Final Truth: The Man You Want to Be Already Has These Habits

He's not debating them.
He's not negotiating with his mood.
He's just doing them because they're part of who he is.

**So here's the real challenge:**

Are you still pretending you'll change when you feel like it?

Or are you ready to build habits so baked into your DNA, skipping them feels weird?

Because if not, keep waiting for that perfect morning where you're "ready."

I'll be over here (on your dusty bookshelf) watching someone else *lap you with discipline.*

# PART II: MONEY & MEANING
## Actually Getting Ahead

Money. And why you still suck at it.

*Money & Meaning*—and no, you can't manifest wealth if you're still making minimum payments on your mental bandwidth.

Ready?

You need a job. You want a purpose. Here's how not to hate both.

Let's start stomping around in the mud where men *actually* drown—money.

Because no one taught you jack except how to get a paycheck and maybe Venmo for pizza.

Let's make you dangerous in the bank account department.

# CHAPTER 5: Career vs. Calling

*Or: How to Not Hate Your Life Between 9 am and Retirement*

Let's face it. You want money.
You want freedom.
You want to wake up and not feel like you're auditioning for a toothpaste commercial where you hate your boss and your soul is trying to crawl out of your eyes.

**Welcome to the postmodern man's dilemma:**

"Should I chase my purpose... or just shut up and pay my bills?"

**Here's the twist:**
You can do both—but not if you confuse them.

The False Binary: Job = Prison, Passion = Salvation

**Some guru on YouTube told you:**
"If you're not making six figures doing what you love by 30, you've failed."

That's nonsense, written by a 24-year-old whose only asset is a rented Audi and a Wi-Fi connection in Bali.

The truth?

Your job is your economic engine.
Your calling is your existential compass.
Confuse them, and you'll crash both.

## What a Career Is *Actually* For

Let's demystify it.

**A good career:**

Pays your rent

Builds marketable skills

Introduces you to people who *aren't* online clowns

Makes you harder to kill in the marketplace

Funds your purpose—until your purpose funds you

"The purpose of a job is freedom, not identity."
—Probably Marcus Aurelius if he had Slack

## But What About Passion?

Yes, you need meaning.
Yes, you need to feel like what you do *matters*.

But meaning without money is a poem.
And you can't pay for therapy with a haiku about your dream.

**So here's the secret weapon**:

You don't find your calling.
You build it.

Like a side project you care about more than scrolling Reddit at work.

## Strategy: Stack Skill + Service + Self

**Here's a simple Venn diagram made of testosterone and realism:**

What you're good at
(Skills that companies/clients will pay for)

What actually helps people
(Think: service, not personal branding with soft lighting)

What makes you feel alive when no one's watching
(This ain't about applause)

The overlap? That's your calling.
Not your fantasy.
Not your Instagram bio.

Your calling is what pulls you forward even when you're tired. And your career is what keeps the lights on until it does.

## And If You Hate Your Job?

**Then here's your reality:**

Use it to fund the next thing

Learn what not to tolerate

Practice discipline in a hard place

Don't die there

"Your job is not your sentence. It's your training camp."
—Graham, whispering from a metaphorical mountaintop

If your boss sucks, learn leadership by contrast.
If your team is lazy, build elite habits in enemy territory.
If you feel stuck, then plan your damn exit.

But don't spiral.
Build.

## Mindset Shift: Stop Looking for "The One"

You don't marry your first job.
You evolve. You adapt. You learn skills and move on.

"You are not your job title. You are your results."
—Tate, probably shirtless but correct again

You want calling? Cool.
Then start solving problems bigger than your own ego.
That's where fulfillment lives. Not in your résumé font.

## Tactical Moves Starting Now

Define your top 5 skills. Not hopes. Skills.

Acknowledge 3 types of problems you'd pay someone to fix.

Find the overlap. Start doing it—even if no one's paying you yet.

In your day job? Become the guy they can't fire. Learn everything. Document it.

Outside of work? Build the next ladder. Slowly. Relentlessly. No whining.

## Final Thought: You're Not Meant to Be Comfortable

You're meant to contribute. To build. To create something so valuable it echoes when you're gone.

But that doesn't mean quitting your job tomorrow and "trusting the universe." That's just romanticized bankruptcy.

**Instead:**

Work the day shift like a soldier. Work your calling like a priest. Merge them when they're both strong enough.

Until then?
No more whining about passion. Get excellent.

# CHAPTER 6: Financial Literacy for Former Boys

*Or: Stop Being Poor... Strategically*

Budgeting, investing, escaping lifestyle creep, and not becoming a 43-year-old with 3 monitors and zero assets.

Grab a metaphorical fork and knife, because this one's protein-packed, debt-crushing, emotionally scarring, and designed to slap the broke mindset out of your skull.

**Spoiler alert:** it's not about crypto or "mindset." It's about how to not be 45 with no assets, five streaming subscriptions, and a drawer full of receipts that all say "DoorDash."

Still hungry? Or need to pace the room first and scream into your career pillow?

If you're over 25 and don't know where your money goes each month, you're not "bad with finances." You're just still thinking like a teenager who believes pizza and overdraft fees are part of God's plan.

This chapter?
It's not "How to Get Rich."
It's How to Stop Being Financially Embarrassing.

## Why You Suck at Money

No one taught you.
School gave you the Pythagorean Theorem but forgot rent, taxes, or how not to die in a mountain of interest.

**Your parents either:**

Avoided money talk like it was nuclear

Or made you think "being rich" meant "being evil"

Or worse—used money to flex instead of educate

So now? You're 33 with 7 different streaming services, no budget, $600 in the bank, and a closet full of "aspirational fashion" you wore twice.

But hey—you "invested in yourself," right?

"Don't mistake consumption for self-improvement."
—Probably Marcus Aurelius, before unsubscribing from HBO Max

## Real Men Budget

No, budgeting isn't "restrictive."
It's literally telling your money what to do instead of letting it vanish like your 20s.

**Here's how to actually budget without becoming a spreadsheet monk:**

The Rule of 60/20/20

60% Needs → Rent, groceries, transportation, therapy (please)

20% Freedom → Stuff you enjoy guilt-free (yes, beer counts)

20% Growth → Saving, investing, paying off debt

Don't like those numbers? Fine. Adjust.

But if you don't know your percentages, you're just vibing financially—and that's how broke people live forever.

## Cut the Lifestyle Creep

You got a raise. Congrats.
Now stop acting like you won the lottery.

More income ≠ more spending.
It just means more *responsibility* and fewer excuses.

That new car?
Cool. But if it's got 22-inch rims and you can't pay your phone bill without Venmo'ing your cousin… we have a problem.

You don't need more money.
You need fewer dumb decisions.

"Wealth isn't what you buy. It's what you *keep.*"
—Napoleon Hill, screaming from the Great Depression

## Debt: The Slow Death

Let's talk about debt because you're probably carrying some.

**Here's the deal:**

Student loans? Not your fault, but they're still yours.

Credit cards? Legalized robbery with your signature on it.

"Buy Now Pay Later"? That's just you saying, "I'm broke today AND tomorrow."

**Tactic:**

Pay off the highest interest stuff first.

Freeze the cards you can't handle like they're evil horcruxes.

Track every cent like it owes you child support.

"A man in debt is not free. He's just a wage slave with Wi-Fi."
—Christopher Graham, probably while unsubscribing from society

## Investing for the Attention-Impaired

You don't need to become a crypto wizard or day-trading monkey.

**Start here:**

Open a Roth IRA (or equivalent wherever you live)

Auto-invest a fixed amount monthly

Buy index funds. Boring. Proven. Grown-up.

Let compound interest do the heavy lifting while you build your empire

"If you're not making money while you sleep, you'll work till you die."
—Warren Buffett, literal grandpa of discipline

## Your Toolkit for Wealth Like a Grown Man

Budget App – Stop winging it. Use something like YNAB or EveryDollar.

Emergency Fund – 3-6 months of expenses. No, your sneaker collection doesn't count.

Track Net Worth – Know your number. Don't fear the truth—fix it.

Automate Everything – Bills, investments, savings. Manual = forgettable.

## One Last Thing: Money is Power—Don't Be Powerless

This isn't about flexing.

**It's about:**

Buying back your time

Helping your family

Sleeping at night without calculating overdraft fees

Not becoming "that guy" who's 45, divorced, and still doesn't own socks without holes

You don't need to become a millionaire (yet).
You need to become competent.

Because the world doesn't care about your good intentions.

Every man speaks. Every man promises. But when the fire comes, the only question is this: can you write the check, and have you built the life, the discipline, and the grit to see it honored?

# CHAPTER 7: Tech, Tools & Boundaries

*"Your Phone Is Not Your Boss, Your Therapist, or Your Girlfriend"*

Boom. Buckle up, because this one is going to rip the power cord straight out of your looped life.

Let's unfuck the relationship with your devices.

## Tech, Tools & Boundaries

You're not "busy," your phone is just your boss. Take back your time and brain space.

**Here it comes—*raw, wired, and fed up with your screen time stats*.**

No one is as productive as they pretend to be when they're staring into their phone like it's a dying Tamagotchi. You're not building a legacy—you're just doomscrolling until your eyeballs start to dry out like old grapes.

We have mistaken *availability* for *value*. If someone texts you, you're expected to respond instantly. If your calendar doesn't have 47 color-coded blocks, you're apparently not ambitious. If you didn't answer a Slack message at 10:13 p.m., you must hate the team.

You're not a man anymore. You're a modem with a beard.

## Your Phone Is Not Your Boss

Stop letting an overpriced rectangle in your pocket dictate the pace of your day. Notifications aren't invitations. They're digital landmines—attention bombs that blow up your focus 47 times a day.

Jordan Peterson didn't say, "Clean your room, and then check your email 32 times before breakfast."

McRaven didn't write *Make Your Bed, Then Open Instagram Reels Until Your Soul Collapses*.

## Your Phone Is Not Your Therapist

You feel stressed, lonely, anxious... and your first instinct is to unlock your phone.

**Congratulations, you've been trained like a lab rat.**

Here's the twist: scrolling isn't self-soothing. It's self-fragmenting.

Villette H. White would call it "mental misalignment through addictive attention loops." Peterson would call it "voluntary chaos." We call it: you need a walk, not a Wi-Fi signal.

## Your Phone Is Not Your Girlfriend

Unless you're dating ChatGPT, in which case—get help. Immediately.

Your screen is not a relationship. That thirst trap on TikTok isn't smiling *at you*. The semi you get when someone hearts your story? Mental masturbation. Empty calories. And you're starving for something real.

If you're checking your phone more than you check in with actual people, you've been seduced by *proximity theatre*. Close, but not connected. Surrounded, but alone.

## Tools, Not Chains

This isn't an anti-tech tantrum. It's a reframe.

Use your phone like a power tool. Pick it up with purpose. Put it down with finality.

Apps don't get to interrupt you. Texts don't get instant loyalty. Work doesn't get 24/7 access to your nervous system.

Your attention is not a community garden. It's a fortress. Guard the damn gate.

## Tactical Moves:

Set app timers for social media. Not "just in case." Because you have the self-control of a sleep-deprived squirrel.

Kill notifications like you're playing whack-a-mole. Leave only essentials—texts, calls, and calendar.

Phone-free mornings until after your morning ritual. You don't need memes before mindfulness.

One screen at a time. If you're watching TV while on your phone while checking your laptop, you're not multitasking—you're malfunctioning.

Tech Sabbath. One day a week. No screens. Just nature, books, weights, and human interaction. (Terrifying, I know.)

You're not addicted to your phone.
You're addicted to *not feeling bored*.

But guess where focus, discipline, and clarity come from?

That's right. Boredom. Stillness. Discomfort. Silence.

And ironically, those things are what make you sharp enough to build the life you're trying to distract yourself from not having.

Unplug. Rewire. Build like a man.

# CHAPTER 8: The Side Hustle Trap

*When "Grind" Becomes a Scam You Pulled on Yourself*

There's something slick and seductive about the phrase *"side hustle."* It sounds gritty. Noble. Like you're out here refusing to be chained to the cubicle wasteland, chasing dreams with fire in your eyes and freedom in your browser tabs.

But let's cut the crap.
The word **"hustle" has always meant scam.**
Not "hard work." Not "entrepreneurial grind." Not "get after it."
**It meant trick. Con. Fraud.**

A pool hustler didn't win because he was talented. He **played you**.

A street hustle wasn't ambition—it was **survival theater**, baiting you into parting with your cash.

And today? That same word is being sprayed with motivational Febreze and sold back to you as a lifestyle.

But *hustle* hasn't changed. You're either **scamming someone**, or **you're being scammed**. Sometimes both. And too often?

**You're scamming yourself.**

You're not building an empire. You're bleeding hours into a Canva template, praying for an algorithmic miracle, and calling it "launching your brand."
You started a business when what you needed was a budget. You bought a domain before you built a backbone. You're spinning a dozen plates labeled "passive income" while your actual life is cracking in half from the weight of all the pretending.

Let's be clear: **a side hustle is inherently bad.** When you're doing it out of fear instead of clarity, it's a hustle. It's a **side con**—and *you're the mark*.

The *hustle mentality* is a lie dressed in productivity drag.

**It tells you:**
– Don't sleep.
– Don't rest.
– Don't feel.
– Keep working or you'll fall behind.

It tells you that your worth is directly tied to how many things you're "building," even if those things are just bloated to-do lists that help you avoid actual growth.

So, if your "freedom plan" feels more like a **digital prison**—with less money, more stress, and the health plan of a Victorian chimney sweep—you didn't escape the system. You just built a shinier version and locked yourself inside it.

That's not ambition.
That's self-inflicted wage slavery with a better font.

So yeah, it's time to audit the grind.

**Ask yourself: Are you building something real—or are you just hustling yourself into burnout with a logo on it?**

Because a scam, no matter how well-branded, is still a scam. Even if the sucker is staring at you from the mirror.

**Let's fix that.**

## The Problem:

- "Hustle" originally meant scam, fraud, or con.
- Hustle culture rebranded panic as purpose.
- You're not building an empire—you're building anxiety with a logo.

## The Real Questions:

- Are you passionate, or just panicked?
- Are you building, or avoiding stillness?
- Do you own the business—or does it own your evenings, weekends, and dignity?

Tactical Fixes:

- **Audit your side business.** Is it profitable, scalable, and purposeful? Or just busywork?

- **Not everything needs a profit model.** Some hobbies are just hobbies. Let them live.

- **Stop grinding in the dark.** Strategy > effort. More spinning doesn't mean more progress.

- **Take a job if you need one.** Stability isn't weakness. Burnout isn't a badge of honor.

- **Focus on skill stacking, not brand stacking.** Be dangerous in your field, not just on your feed.

If your "freedom plan" makes you anxious, broke, and exhausted, you didn't escape the rat race—you are side-hustling yourself.

# PART III: PEOPLE & POWER
## How Not to Be a Weird Island

## CHAPTER 9: Male Friendships – The Vanishing Species

*"Group Chats Are Not Brotherhood"*

Why do you have group chats but no one to call when you're in a crisis? Rebuilding your social skeleton.

Look, I get it. You're "busy."

You've got a job, a podcast queue, a side hustle that's mostly just Googling how to start a side hustle, and maybe a relationship if the stars align and your phone battery doesn't die at the wrong time.

**But let me ask you something gut-level honest:**

When's the last time you sat across from another man, looked him in the eye, and talked about something real?
(And no, "bro this protein powder slaps" doesn't count.)

## The Crisis of Connection

Modern male friendship has gone the way of the dad bod—soft, passive, and increasingly optional.

You *like* your friends' posts.

You *LOL* in the group chat.

You *may see each other a couple of* times a year... if nobody flakes and the stars align, and someone's wife doesn't schedule a surprise trip to a crystal healing retreat.

What we've built is not a brotherhood. It's a digital holding cell full of punchlines, sports takes, and emotional constipation.

You're not connected. You're just accessible.

## Why It Hurts (Even If You Don't Feel It Yet)

Peterson would say this is chaos disguised as comfort.

Christopher Graham might call it spiritual atrophy.

And your gut—if you actually sat with it—would probably just mutter,

"Yeah... this ain't it."

Men need men. Not in a weird cult sauna-circle kind of way.

In a steel-sharpening-steel, punch-each-others ' egos-back-into-shape kind of way.

You need the guy who sees through your bullshit.

The guy who tells you you're drifting.

The guy who shows up when you're face-down in your own mess.

And that guy? Doesn't materialize by accident. You have to build him.

Which means you have to show up too.

## Tactical Reconnection

Let's get practical. No incense. No group hugs (unless you're into that, no shame).

**Just a few things to start building your brotherhood again:**

Schedule standing meetups. Coffee. Gym. Walks. Set it. Protect it. Repeat.

Do hard things together. Train. Compete. Volunteer. Build something. Struggle side-by-side.

Ask better questions. "What's been heavy lately?" hits harder than "What's new?"

Don't disappear when life gets good. That's when most guys ghost their crew. Be the one who stays.

## Real Talk: Brotherhood Is Grit, Not Vibes

Friendship isn't convenient. It's a decision.
It's following up, showing up, and calling a man when he goes silent.

And letting him do the same for you—even when your ego's bruised.

Because when the marriage shakes, the job falls apart, or you're just spiraling at 2 am with no answers—you don't need another YouTube video.

You need *him*.
And *he* needs *you*.

So close the app. Call your people.
Make friendship a ritual again—not just a reaction.

# CHAPTER 10: Dating, Partnership & not being a Clown

You might want to stretch first. It's about to get emotionally athletic.

Dating, Partnership, and Not Being a Clown Modern relationships decoded. Learn to apologize like you mean it.

*Stop Self-Sabotaging & Learn to Apologize Without Crying Into a Hoodie*

**Let's not sugarcoat it:** modern dating is a minefield covered in emojis, ghosting, and guys who think emotional intelligence means asking "u up?" with slightly more eye contact.

And you? You're not immune.

You want connection. You want sex. You want to feel seen and respected.

**But what you *do* is:**

Swipe yourself into oblivion.

Reply with a fire emoji instead of a complete sentence.

Bail on anything that smells like emotional risk.

Congrats, you're now emotionally malnourished, romantically confused, and pretending memes are intimacy.

## Why You Suck at This (It's Not Entirely Your Fault)

Let's be fair. You weren't trained for this.

Your dad didn't teach you how to navigate modern emotional terrain. School didn't teach you what healthy vulnerability looks like. The internet told you to be either a simp or an alpha, with nothing in between.

Christopher Graham would call this "emotional outsourcing." You gave your emotional literacy to culture—and it gave you TikToks and Tinder.

Peterson's take? You need order, structure, and responsibility. Not another hookup. A *mission* for your heart, not just your libido.

But don't worry. We're not turning this into a therapy circle with scented candles. We're just going to clean up your act, so you stop being a walking red flag with a Spotify playlist.

## First, Let's Talk About Self-Sabotage

You're great at the chase. Terrible at the keep. You get anxious when it's going too well. You disappear instead of speaking up. You manufacture drama just to feel something.

That's not masculinity. That's insecurity doing push-ups in your head.

Stop dating people you want to fix.

Stop hiding behind sarcasm when things get real.

Stop pretending detachment is power.

Attachment isn't a weakness. It's what makes you human.

## Also: You Don't Communicate, You Telepath

"I thought she knew."

"She should've picked up on the vibe."

"My silence meant I was thinking."

NOPE. None of that holds up in court, champ.

You have to speak. Say what you feel. Risk being wrong. Own your confusion.

Because guess what? Avoiding emotional messes just makes bigger ones.

Villette White would tell you that unspoken thought becomes unformed energy—and unformed energy becomes inner chaos.

Speak. Feel. Clarify. Rinse. Repeat.

## How to Clean Up the Relationship Mess

Stop leading with image. Show up with *substance*, not just "look at my perfect curated life."

Apologize like a man. That means no "I'm sorry *you feel that way*." Take the hit when you screw up. Then fix it.

Talk early. Don't let resentment ferment into passive-aggressive soup.

Don't ghost. That's what cowards do. And we're building warriors, remember?

Respect boundaries. Hers, yours, reality's.

## Real Partnership Is Work (And That's the Point)

Relationships aren't supposed to be easy. They're supposed to be *worth it*.

You show up.
You get uncomfortable.
You deal with your triggers instead of defending them.
You love like it's a practice—not a performance.

Because otherwise? You're just another guy yelling "women don't want nice guys anymore" into the void while dodging accountability like it's cardio.

## One-Liner to Tattoo on Your Brain:

"Don't build a life so lonely that even success feels like failure."

# CHAPTER 11: Leadership without too much Ego

Time to learn how to lead without being a dictator in a fitted polo.

In your work, community, or family. Less "alpha male", more "actual adult who can manage conflict."

*You're Not the Main Character, But You Are the Guide*

### Let's get one thing out of the way:

If you still think leadership means barking orders and flexing in front of a whiteboard, this chapter is going to hurt.

Authentic leadership isn't about dominance. It's about *direction*. It's not the loudest voice—it's the *clearest*. It's not charisma—it's *consistency*.

But you were never taught that, were you?

### You were handed two leadership templates:

*The Alpha Gorilla:* Loud, angry, chest-thumping power tripper.

*The Passive Boss:* Shrugging his way through life while the team burns out.

*Spoiler alert:* both of those suck.

You don't need a script. You need a spine. And maybe a system that doesn't rely on caffeine, intimidation, or pretending to be Tony Robbins on creatine.

## Who Put You in Charge? (And Why That Matters)

Peterson would tell you that leadership starts with cleaning your damn room. And he's right.

Christopher Graham would say it's about becoming the King archetype—not to rule, but to *serve with vision*.

McRaven would shout something about accountability and excellence in the same breath, probably while doing push-ups.

*Here's the throughline:* If you can't lead yourself, you can't lead anyone else.

And no, that doesn't mean being perfect. It means showing up—even when it sucks.

**Especially when it sucks.**

## What Real Leadership Looks Like

It's boring.

Not glamorous.

Not viral.

Just *relentless responsibility*.

It's clear. Say what you mean. Mean what you say. No riddles, no vibes.

It's vulnerable. Not weepy TED talk vulnerability. Just the courage to admit when you're out of your depth—and ask for help.

It's personal. Know your people. Don't just manage them—mentor them.

It's duplicatable. If your system falls apart without you, you're not a leader—you're a bottleneck.

## Ego Is the Hidden Enemy

Your ego wants credit. Applause. Power. But leadership isn't about being the hero.

It's about being the guide. The *bridge*. The *anchor*.

Donald Trump (yes, really) says in *The Art of the Deal*: "I like thinking big. I always have."

That's fine—but the *biggest* thinkers know when to shut up and *listen*.

If you're always the smartest guy in the room, you're in the wrong room—or you've silenced everyone else.

## Tactical Leadership for Real Life

*Whether you're running a team, a family, or just yourself:*

Set the tone. The vibe starts with you. If you're chaotic, everyone else will be too.

Make decisions. Don't hide in ambiguity. Pick a direction and adjust later.

Accept the blame, share the credit. If it fails, it's on you. If it wins, shine the light on others.

Create systems, not dependencies. Build people who can build without you.

Speak last. Let others share first. Then bring clarity, not noise.

## Final Gut Punch

Authentic leaders aren't idolized.
They're *trusted*.

They don't *demand* respect. They *earn* it—by showing up, standing firm, and lifting others while they carry the weight.

So stop chasing "alpha" energy and start cultivating *king energy*.
The world has enough influencers.
We need builders. Mentors. Anchors.

The kind of men who don't just lead.
They *last*.

Added to the eternal gospel of Not Being a Coward. Here's where it belongs—right in the next *Shi*t No One Told Me* installment under "Honor Isn't Situational (You Just Keep Failing the Test)".

Don't throw your buddy under the bus for a woman. It's weak, and she'll smell it. Loyalty matters. If your friendship gets tossed just because she made a face, you weren't a friend—you were a temporary roommate in manhood.

Also? Don't throw a woman under the bus for a buddy. That's not loyalty—it's cowardice hiding behind the boys' club. Being a man means protecting the truth, not just the team.

If you need to betray someone to feel powerful, you're not a man.

You're just a traitor with a gym membership.

# CHAPTER 12: Legacy, not just Income

*"You Can't Take Your Crypto Wallet to the Grave"*

What will your life actually *mean*? Because you can't take your crypto wallet to the grave.

Let's get existential for a second. Not soft. Not sentimental. Just real.

**You're going to die.**

Probably not today (unless you're reading this while doing something stupid), but eventually, the lights go out. And when they do? Nobody's reading your bank statement at your funeral.

They're talking about what kind of man you were.

How you showed up. What you built. Who you lifted.

Legacy isn't what you leave behind. It's what you live out—loud, daily, and with intention.

## What the Greats Say (And Why It's Not Just Philosophy Bullshit)

**Peterson:** "Pick up the heaviest thing you can carry and carry it." Why? Because burden breeds meaning.

**Graham:** Your hero's journey doesn't end when you win—it ends when you *give back*.

**Napoleon Hill:** You don't just think and grow rich—you think, grow, and *teach*.

**Marcus Aurelius:** "What we do now echoes in eternity." (Yes, *Gladiator* ripped that. Still true.)

You are not your income. You are your *impact*.

## So What Are You Actually Building?

**Ask yourself:** If you died next week, what's unfinished that actually *matters*?

Who's better off because they knew you?

Would your son know how to be a man because you showed him—or would he have to Google it? Or buy a book?

You don't need to start a foundation. Just start *acting like your life means something bigger than your calendar app and fantasy football league.*

## Work Is Not Your Legacy (But It's Part of It)

You work hard. Great. But *why*?

To buy things? To prove something to people who don't care? To fill the God-shaped hole with another Amazon package?

**Here's the twist:** Work is sacred—when it *serves, when* it builds, when it multiplies value beyond just your wallet.

Teach. Mentor. Model. Leave blueprints, not breadcrumbs.

**Villette White:** The untrained mind creates only for self. The trained mind *creates for generations*.

## You're the Ancestor Now

One day, someone will trace their strength back to you. Not because you posted a reel with motivational music, but because you *walked the walk*.

You listened. You endured. You spoke truth when it was inconvenient. You led when no one else would. You didn't flinch.

Income is what you make. Legacy is what you make *matter*.

One fades with inflation—the other compounds across lifetimes.

You get to choose. So... what's your next move?

# OUTRO: Becoming Dangerous

*"Because the World Doesn't Need More Passive Men. It Needs Builders With Teeth."*

Let's land this warship.

You've just walked through 12 chapters of systems, sanity, grit, fire, masculinity, legacy, and calling your own damn bluff.

If your nervous system isn't at least mildly electrified, check your pulse or go back to Chapter 1 and read it again *like you mean it*.

Ah, yes. The **mic drop** version. The one that makes the reader close the book slowly, sit in stunned silence, and whisper something like, *"...shit."*

If you made it here, you've the slap. Now comes the test. Because *reading* this book doesn't mean a damn thing. Not unless it gets under your skin and rewires your spine.

You don't need to feel inspired. You need to feel **responsible.** Responsible for the way you show up. For how you spend your time, your energy, your name. For the standards you've either enforced or abandoned.

This isn't the part where I say, "You got this."
This is where I say: *stop acting like someone else is going to do it for you.*

You don't get to blame the algorithm, your upbringing, or the culture.

You're grown. You have hands. A brain. A calendar. You've been given the tools. Use them—or stay behind.

**And let's be clear:**
If you walk away from this book and immediately start calling strangers *"brother"*...
You didn't get it.

Brotherhood is *earned*. Through presence. Through pain. Through proof. Not through hashtags or hollow handshakes.

**Also:** if you find yourself casually throwing around *"dude"* like a nervous tic, stop. That word is a warning. Use it when someone's acting out of pocket—**including yourself.**

**Sometimes the man in the mirror needs to be told:** "Get it together, dude."

Being a man is about discernment. Knowing when to throw a punch—verbally, spiritually, emotionally— And knowing when to walk away without looking weak.

**Zen isn't silence.** Zen is power with precision. It's calm so deep it can afford to be sharp.

Your legacy doesn't start when you're rich. It starts when you take responsibility for every action, every word, every moment from here forward.

**So no more:**

- Waiting until you "feel ready."
- Hoping the perfect job, woman, or answer shows up.
- Cosplaying masculinity with quotes and gear but no grit.

Now is the moment. This is the fork in the road.

Walk one way, and you go back to sleep—with better vocabulary but the same soft habits.

Walk the other?

**You become something terrifying in the best possible way:** A man who knows who he is—and lives like it.

Boom. Page closed. Lights off. Do the work.

# The Grown Man Operating System™

1. **Identity:** Know who you are—without applause.

2. **Mind:** Build the mental fortress first.

3. **Body:** Energy > aesthetics. Train like it matters.

4. **Habits:** Stack don't sprint.

5. **Work:** Purpose + paycheck. One without the other is burnout.

6. **Money:** Use it. Don't worship it.

7. **Tech:** Control it or it controls you.

8. **Friends:** Make some. Be one. Save your damn life.

9. **Love:** Learn intimacy without turning it into a TED Talk.

10. **Leadership:** Less alpha, more anchor.

11. **Legacy:** Play the long game.

12. **Dangerous Goodness:** Scare the weak parts of yourself until they become strong.

# WHAT WE'RE NOT DOING:

## Monthly Action Plans

Because guess what? Life doesn't run on your 30-day spreadsheet. You're not a sales funnel. You're a man with moods, stress, and random Tuesday existential dread. Real growth doesn't happen in neat monthly increments—it happens in *moments of decision*, repeated inconsistently, then adapted like an actual adult. Monthly plans give false comfort. We build systems that flex.

## Habit Tracking Templates

**Let me translate:**

"I did 17 push-ups and flossed. Where's my six-pack and emotional stability?"

Here's the truth—*tracking* doesn't transform. **Doing does.** You don't need to count streaks like a middle school Snapchat addict. You need to become the kind of man who works out because it's who he is, not because his app gave him a gold star.

Track habits if it helps—but don't confuse color-coded charts with character. One is dopamine. The other is discipline.

## Journaling Templates

### "Today I feel..." Oh shut up.

You want to journal? Great. Do it raw. Write as if your future son is reading it. Cry on the page. Rage on the page. But don't force it through some prefab prompt like "3 things I'm grateful for." You're not a Pinterest board. You're a furnace. Burn the page if you have to.

## Meal Plans

Unless you're cutting for a fight, prepping for a bodybuilding show, or dealing with a medical issue, obsessing over grams of quinoa is a fast track to insanity. Eat real food. Eat like a man who needs to build things, lift things, *live long enough to raise kings*.

You don't need a spreadsheet. You need a skillet and some damn discipline.

# WHAT YOU DO INSTEAD:

Wake up and choose forward movement *every day*, not every 30.

Build rituals, not rigid schedules.

Drop the obsession with optimization and pick up the hammer of repetition.

Don't track your habits. Become someone who doesn't negotiate them.

And for the love of iron, *eat like you're fueling a mission*, not surviving a calorie quiz.

# Final word?

Templates are for children.

Transformation is for men.

You want structure? Good.

But we don't do cages. We build castles.

And this? This is the construction site.

# SHIT NO ONE TOLD ME – VOL. 1:
## But Should've

This is where we take off the gloves, drop the therapist voice, and hit you with 50-caliber honesty. Rapid-fire. No sugar, no lube, just facts you should've gotten from a dad, a mentor, or literally *any functioning adult*—but didn't.

• Motivation is a liar. Discipline is your only friend that doesn't flake.

• Nobody cares how you feel until you fix how you act.

• Your abs don't matter. Your character does. But also...train your damn body.

• She doesn't want a prince. She wants a man with a spine, a plan, and actual hygiene.

• If you can't sit alone in silence, you're not strong. You're overstimulated.

• Alcohol isn't a personality. It's anesthesia.

• You're not "behind." You're just undisciplined and distracted.

• You'll never be fully "ready." Start anyway. Start anywhere. Fear doesn't go away. You outgrow it.

- Comfort is the slow death. Growth is the wound that heals into armor.

- If your friends mock your goals, they're not friends—they're anchors.

- You will lose people when you level up. Let them go. Pack light for the next phase.

- Porn is not harmless. It's a slow poison to your confidence, relationships, and brain.

- If your phone is the first and last thing you touch every day, congrats—you're in a relationship with a device that's using you.

- Most "alpha males" online are overcompensating for something that cries at night.

- Stop waiting for permission to become dangerous in a good way.

- Being broke isn't a character flaw. Staying broke on purpose is.

- You don't need to be perfect to be respected—you need to *be consistent*.

- There's no "right time" to leave the wrong job, the wrong woman, or the wrong version of yourself.

- The gym won't fix your soul. But it's a good place to start.

• Therapy isn't a weakness. Ignoring your mental illness while deadlifting is.

• If your dad wasn't a blueprint, become one.

Still breathing? Good.

Print this out. Tape it to your mirror. Or your fridge. Or your steering wheel.
Whatever it takes to remember that you're not broken—you're just building.

# SHIT NO ONE TOLD ME – VOL. 2:

## The Coward List

If you think this makes you a man, you're already lost.

This isn't virtue-signaling. This is a code.
Because there's a difference between *being dangerous* and being *disgusting*.
Here's how you know you've crossed the line from man to coward:

## You Are a Coward If...

• **You hit a woman smaller and weaker than you.**
No. You're not a man. You're a malfunction. Get fixed or stay alone forever.

• **You hit a man *because you think he can't hit back*.**
You're not tough. You're a predator with a low IQ and a worse haircut.

• **You abuse kids—physically, emotionally, sexually, psychologically.**
May your Wi-Fi be slow, your gains plateau, and the law find you fast.

- **You kill giraffes, elephants, lions, or any majestic animal *for sport*.**
Not for survival. Not for food. Just for Instagram. That's not manly—that's sociopathic LARPing.

- **You kick a dog.**
You're the emotional equivalent of unseasoned tofu. A bully in dad shoes. May karma make your pillow hot forever.

- **You leave your pet at home 12 hours a day with no stimulation, affection, or care.**
Then blame the dog for being "bad." You're not alpha. You're just lazy with a superiority complex.

- **You cheat and call it "just being a man."**
No. You're just emotionally underdeveloped and spiritually constipated. Monogamy's not for everyone—but *honesty* is.

- **You record people having meltdowns in public instead of helping.**
Congrats. You've chosen clout over character. Hope your followers visit you in the hospital when *you're* the one breaking down.

- **You mock men for crying, then wonder why suicide rates are higher for us.**
We can grieve and still throw hands.

- **You get women drunk to "hook up easier."**

*Spoiler:* that's not a game. That's coercion wrapped in bad cologne.

- **You call discipline "toxic" and excuses "self-care."**

Guess what? Weakness doesn't age well. It just calcifies.

- **You chase fame and ignore your family.**

Strangers cheering you on while your kid eats dinner alone isn't a flex.

- **You post about protecting women, but can't keep your own ego in check for five minutes.**

Save the hashtags. Start with your reflection.

- **You think "providing" means you don't have to parent.**

Money doesn't replace presence. You don't get extra credit for feeding a kid you never talk to.

- **You quit on your life and blame the world.**

You were given one shot. One frame. Make it count—or step aside for someone who will.

# SHIT NO ONE TOLD ME – VOL. 3:

"How to Know You're Actually Growing (Not Just Rebranding Your Coping Mechanisms)"
*Subtitle: Stop slapping affirmations on your dysfunction and calling it 'healing.'*

## From Christopher Graham (Emotional Transformation Sensei):

In *Falling Down, Growing Up*, Graham says transformation doesn't mean *looking* better—it means *becoming* more self-aware, even when the truth sucks.

"True growth comes from tension, loss, and self-confrontation—not from performative journaling or Instagram therapy quotes."

So no, lighting a sage stick in your emotionally unavailable apartment doesn't mean you're evolving. You're just creating a nice smell for your avoidance to live in.

## From Jordan Peterson (The Shadow Whisperer):

Peterson's big point: Integration > avoidance.

"If you can't acknowledge your capacity for darkness, your light is probably fake."

Translation: If your 'growth' is just smiling more while suppressing rage and people-pleasing yourself into a breakdown, that's not growth. That's a spiritual hostage situation.

## From Villette H. White (Mind Mechanic & Thought Alchemist):

White says the mind must be trained like a muscle—not indulged like a toddler.

"Healing is not passive. It is an active, conscious redirection of thought."

So if you're still blaming "energy vampires" while ghosting responsibility, guess what—you're the vampire. And the meal is your potential.

## From Marcus Aurelius (Stoic Sledgehammer):

"Just because it feels good doesn't mean it's good. And just because it hurts doesn't mean it's bad."

So yeah—growth might *feel* like failure. But so does leg day. That's the point.
Fake growth is dopamine. Real growth is *discipline with meaning*.

## Signs You're Actually Growing:

☑ You call yourself out before others do.

☑ You say, "I was wrong" without it feeling like death.

☑ You choose the hard conversation over the silent grudge.

☑ You do the thing even though you *don't feel like it*.

☑ You stop posting about your "glow up" and just quietly build.

☑ You own your shit without weaponizing your trauma.

## Signs You're Just Rebranding Coping Mechanisms:

✗ You call every breakup a "lesson," but never change your dating patterns.

✗ You say you're "protecting your energy" but really just avoiding accountability.

✗ You confuse busyness with worth.

✗ You slap "healing journey" on every excuse to stay stuck.

✗ You think new crystals = new character.

# INFLUENCERS & FRAMEWORK

*This book didn't spring out of a void. It's a war-forged mixtape of some of the hardest, wisest, and most brutally honest minds across time and space. If anything in here hits you in the chest—it probably came from one of these legends:*

Jordan Peterson *– Archetypes, order, meaning, and personal responsibility (plus an entire rulebook you should've read at 19)*

Admiral William McRaven *– Military discipline, micro-rituals, and systemized toughness that survives chaos*

Christopher Graham *– Hero's journey, masculine evolution, mystical fire-forging of the modern soul*

Napoleon Hill *– Manifestation through desire, clarity, and faith-driven domination of fear*

Villette H. White *– Mental healing, metaphysical alignment, and mindset as your battlefield*

Divine Science (Cramer/James) *– Conscious thought as creative force; the inner world shapes the outer one*

**Andrew Tate** – *No-excuses intensity and aggressive self-command (used strategically, not worshipped blindly)*

**Marcus Aurelius** – *Stoic virtue, unshakeable mental grit, and the quiet power of self-governance*

**Donald J. Trump** – *Tactical negotiation, media judo, and turning boldness into leverage (selectively weaponized from The Art of the Deal)*

# BONUS FEATURES:

### What Now?

You've got the tools. The map. The mission. *So here's the question that matters:*

**Are you about to just highlight this book and shelf it next to the other ones that didn't change a damn thing?**

Or are you going to *live it*—in the quiet, in the chaos, and when no one's watching? This isn't about hype. It's about heat.

It's about showing up when you're tired, uncertain, unmotivated—and doing it anyway.

It's about becoming the kind of man whose habits are louder than his mouth. One who doesn't just *talk legacy*. He leaves one.

Because newsflash: **the world is still on fire.**

And no one's handing out medals for "almost got serious." So now you do the work. Daily. Relentlessly. Without applause. This is the way.

And when you're ready to find out if you're actually walking the walk? Turn to the self-assessment quizzes.

They're mirrors—brutal ones.

# How Solid Is Your Inner Framework?

*(Score yourself 1–5 on each. Be honest. No one's watching. Except your future self.)*

## MINDSET & PHILOSOPHY (Peterson, White, Aurelius)

I take full responsibility for my choices—even the dumb ones.

I know what I believe in—and why.

I can suffer without blaming the world for it.

I track negative thinking like I'd track a virus in my system.

I don't need chaos to feel alive.

## HABITS & DISCIPLINE (McRaven, Trump, Hill)

My morning has structure, not just coffee and chaos.

I do hard things, especially when I don't want to.

I finish what I start—even when it sucks.

I have financial discipline (budgeting, investing, not being a goldfish with money).

I don't wait for motivation. I move anyway.

## IDENTITY & DIRECTION (Graham, Tate, Divine Science)

I know what "success" means *for me*—not Instagram.

I've questioned my old stories—and written better ones.

I feel dangerous in a good way: controlled power.

I'm building something bigger than my ego.

I live by design, not default.

## RELATIONSHIPS & LEGACY (Hill, Graham, Aurelius)

I show up for my people when it counts.

I lead with integrity, not ego.

I've got male friendships that go deeper than fantasy football.

I'm becoming someone I'd want my kids to model— even if I don't have kids.

My legacy matters more to me than my likes.

## RESULTS:

### 21–30: LIMP FRAME

You've got potential, but you're operating like a discount IKEA bookshelf. Wobbly. Start with systems. Chapter 1 is calling you.

### 31–50: DUCT-TAPED MAN

You're doing stuff right, but it's holding together with hustle, hope, and Red Bull—time to upgrade to steel-beam foundations.

### 51–70: BUILDER STATUS

You're showing up, putting in reps, and not bullshitting yourself. Stay sharp, and don't coast. You're not done.

### 71–80: DANGEROUS IN A GOOD WAY

You're what this book is about. Keep building. Now go drag three other men with you.

## ARE YOU ADDICTED TO COMFORT?

*(Score yourself 1–5: 1 = Nope, 5 = Help.)*

## COMFORT CREEP

I hit snooze more than I hit goals.

If something feels uncomfortable, I avoid it. Automatically.

My free time looks like a cross between Netflix, snacks, and numbness.

I fantasize about results, but fear the effort.

My version of risk is ordering the spicy option at Chipotle.

## DISCIPLINE DODGING

I skip workouts with the excuse of "listening to my body." (Translation: I'm lazy.)

I have more Amazon boxes than completed projects.

I read about habits more than I actually build them.

I wait for "motivation" instead of creating momentum.

I bail when things stop being "fun."

## FALSE SECURITY

I avoid confrontation—even when I know I should speak up.

I numb myself with food, scrolling, or busywork when things get real.

I fear failure more than I crave success.

I'd rather be *liked* than *respected*.

I confuse peace with passivity.

## RESULTS:

### 15–25: COMFORT MONK

You've mastered the art of sedation. You're not resting—you're rusting. The world doesn't need another man on emotional melatonin. It requires you to be awake. Start by doing something that sucks—on purpose.

### 26–45: BUBBLE WRAPPED

You're trying. Sort of. But comfort has you in a chokehold disguised as self-care—time to stop pampering your fear and start disciplining your edge. Turn to Chapter 3 and let's get physical.

### 46–60: EDGE RUNNER

You understand the value of discomfort—but you still flinch. Good. Now do it anyway. Comfort is a liar with soft hands. You're stronger than you think.

### 61–75: FIREWALKER

You don't run from pressure. You train under it. You're not comfort's slave—you use it as fuel. You're dangerous in the best way. Just don't get cocky. You know what happens to guys who stop sharpening their blades.

## THE EMOTIONAL STRENGTH TEST: ARE YOU JUST STOIC, OR ACTUALLY STRONG?

*(Rate each 1–5. Be honest. That's the whole point.)*

## TRUE STRENGTH

I can admit when I'm wrong—without shrinking.

I express anger without turning into a toddler or a tyrant.

I let people in without losing myself.

I don't need to be "right"—I need to grow.

I handle rejection without spiraling into doom scrolls or Doritos.

## FAKE STOICISM

I pretend I'm fine instead of dealing with what's real.

I've mastered the art of the "I'm good" lie.

I call emotional people weak to avoid my own feelings.

I use logic as a weapon, not a tool.

I avoid having hard conversations instead of confronting people.

## EMOTIONAL INTELLIGENCE

I know what I'm feeling—and why.

I don't expect others to read my mind.

I sit with uncomfortable emotions without trying to escape them.

I can validate others without invalidating myself.

I'm not afraid of therapy. I'm afraid of staying stuck.

RESULTS:

### 15–25: EMOTIONAL DODGER
You've got the emotional vocabulary of a broken vending machine. Either nothing comes out, or it's just anger-flavored sadness. This isn't stoicism—it's shutdown—time to reboot.

### 26–45: STRENGTH IN PROGRESS
You're catching yourself and feeling more and talking less bullshit. That's real growth. Stay with it. It's awkward, vulnerable, and worth it.

### 46–60: THE BALANCED MAN
You're not reactive. You're responsive. You're not cold. You're composed. And guess what? That makes you dangerous in the best damn way.

### 61–75: UNFUCKWITHABLE
You feel deep. You lead hard. You stay grounded. Emotional strength isn't about silence—it's about mastery. You don't just survive storms. You steer ships through them.

## YOUR PHONE IS NOT YOUR THERAPIST: A DIGITAL DETOX DIAGNOSIS

*(Rate 1–5, then ... put your phone down.)*

### DIGITAL DEPENDENCY

I check my phone before I pee in the morning.

If I leave the house without it, I panic like I forgot a kidney.

My screen time is higher than my confidence.

I scroll when I'm bored, stressed, lonely, or hungry.

I've caught myself doomscrolling in the middle of a "deep convo."

### ATTENTION FRACTURE

I can't watch a movie without checking my phone.

I interrupt workouts, conversations, or sleep... for notifications.

I reply faster to DMs than I do to my own goals.

I've read more comment sections than actual books this year.

I have multiple apps to "relax" and they all make me tense.

### DIGITAL DISCIPLINE

I schedule phone-free time—intentionally.

I use tech. It doesn't use me.

I can go hours without a dopamine hit.

I've uninstalled apps that hijack my focus.

I spend more time creating than consuming.

## RESULTS:

### 15–25: WALKING NOTIFICATION CENTER

You're not living life. You're reacting to it—one buzz at a time. You're not addicted. You're conditioned. And you can change it. Chapter 8 was literally written to drag you out of this.

### 26–45: DISTRACTED, BUT AWARE

You're starting to notice your patterns—and that's power. Keep reclaiming space. You don't need to delete everything. Just stop letting your phone parent you.

### 46–60: SCREEN SHAMAN

You're in control. Tech is your tool, not your tyrant. You're not addicted to noise. You're addicted to progress. And that's rare.

### 61–75: RARE SPECIMEN

You probably wrote this quiz. Either that or you live in a cabin and crush raw liver for breakfast. You're thriving off the grid. The rest of us are trying to catch up.

# FURTHER READING

## You're Not a Moron, You're Just Underequipped

Congratulations. If you made it this far, you're either serious about changing your life or too stubborn to admit you need a nap. Either way, here's the "next layer"—the books that helped build this beast. You won't need incense or a vision board: just a pen, a brain, and a reason.

## 12 *Rules for Life* – Jordan B. Peterson

**Read it:** You've been avoiding discipline by calling yourself "creative."
**What it delivers:** Order. Depth. The psychological blueprint for not being a mess. Also lobsters.

## *Make Your Bed* – Admiral William H. McRaven

**Read it:** You think motivation is enough.
**What it delivers:** Bite-sized discipline that doesn't care about your feelings. Military logic for civilian chaos.

### 100 Things Everyone Should Know – Christopher Graham

**Read it:** You're convinced life should've come with a manual.
**What it delivers:** Plainspoken, punchy truth. Think of it like your wise uncle yelling life wisdom at you from the garage.

### Falling Down, Growing Up – Christopher Graham

**Read it:** You're a man who's been knocked down and is tired of pretending it didn't hurt.
**What it delivers:** Emotional evolution, masculine rebirth, and the real cost of avoiding your own depth.

### The Art of Transformation – Christopher Graham

**Read it:** You're ready to stop performing and actually *transform*.
**What it delivers:** Hypnosis, spirituality, raw psychology—served without a side of New Age fluff.

## Mental Healing Made Easy – Villette H. White

**Read it:** Your brain is your worst roommate.
**What it delivers:** Metaphysical mindset reprogramming. No vibes. Just results.

## Think and Grow Rich – Napoleon Hill

**Read it:** You're broke *and* scattered.
**What it delivers:** Desire → Discipline → Dominance. Plus, a reminder that vague ambition gets you nowhere.

## Divine Science: Its Principle and Practice – Cramer/James

**Read it:** You feel the spiritual itch but don't want to join a cult.
**What it delivers:** Mindset, metaphysics, and the shocking power of focused thought.

## The Art of the Deal – Donald J. Trump

**Read it:** You need to negotiate without crying.
**What it delivers:** Confidence. Strategy. And the occasional gold-plated sentence. Use with caution and a brain.

## Selected Interviews– Andrew Tate

**Read/Listen to it:** You want brutal honesty without the sugar.

**What it delivers:** No-excuse accountability, confidence, and unapologetic focus. Use sparingly. He's the spice, not the steak.

## Meditations/Stoicism – Marcus Aurelius

**Read it:** You're tired of emotional chaos and need a code.

**What it delivers:** Quiet strength. Ancient clarity. No memes, just mastery.

**Buckle up.**

These aren't just reading recs.

These are *warning labels* for your ego.

You asked for brutal honesty, and here it comes like a freight train with no brakes and a bullhorn.